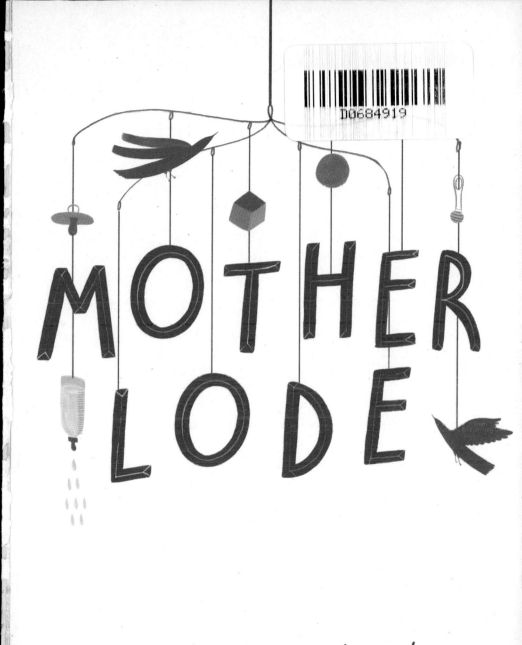

MOTHER LODE

Georgie McAusland

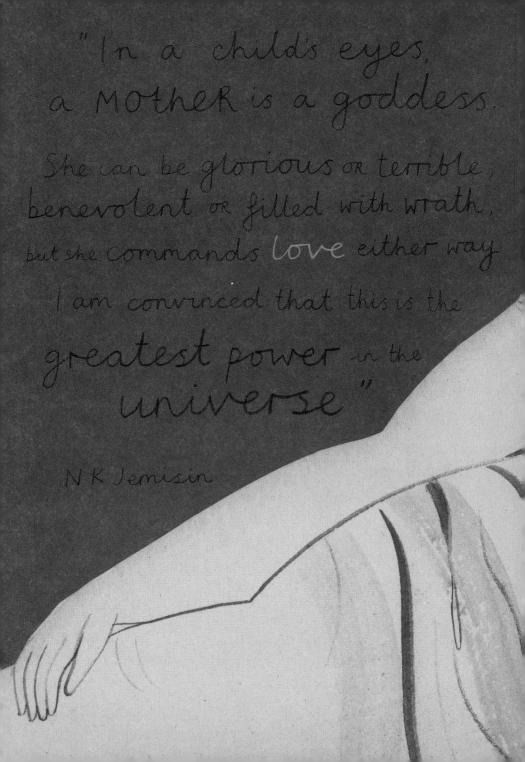

"In a child's eyes,
a MOTHER is a goddess.

She can be glorious or terrible,
benevolent or filled with wrath,
but she commands love either way

I am convinced that this is the

greatest power in the

universe"

N K Jemisin

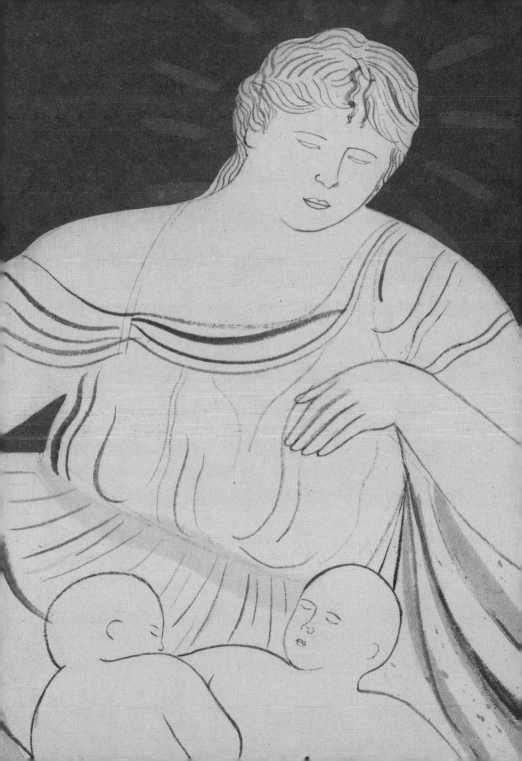

WELCOME

to Motherlode -

the interactive journal in which to explore all the <u>horrors</u> of parenthood without fear of judgement.

Motherhood can be isolating, all our hard-earned adult life skills suddenly rendered insignificant by a hysterical 8 pound tyrant.

The sleep deprivation, crying and the overwhelming sense of guilt and inadequacy...

Is it any wonder we retreat into ourselves, falling back on whatever bizarre coping mechanisms were passed onto us by our own mothers?

So write, draw, doodle and scrawl to your heart's delight - giving expression to some of these experiences can make it all feel more managable.

Plus it will be a hilarious read a few years down the line. Because it will easier and against all odds you will get through it.

The way we were

Write about your life before you were pregnant.
Try to be honest about who you were and what your life was like.

Write about your relationship, your career,
your lifestyle before there was a baby.

"Everything grows rounder and wider and weirder, and I sit here in the middle of it all and wonder who in the world you will turn out to be"

Carrie Fisher

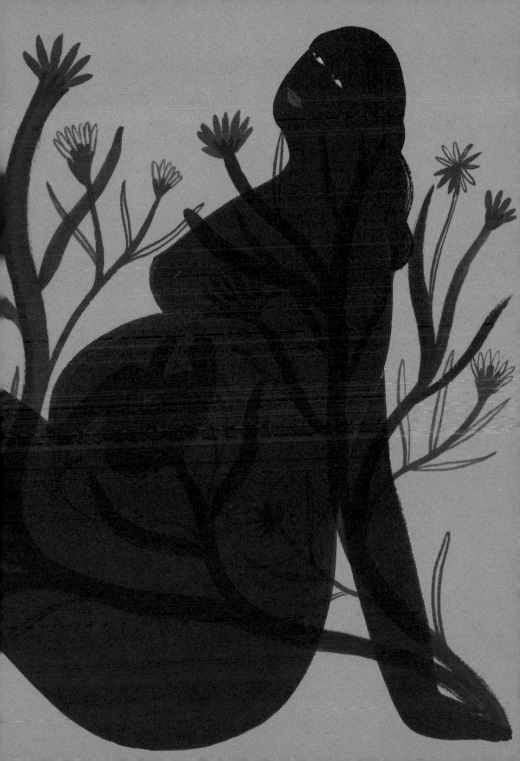

How it happened

Write about the moment you found out you were pregnant. How did you feel? What was the lead up to the pregnancy?

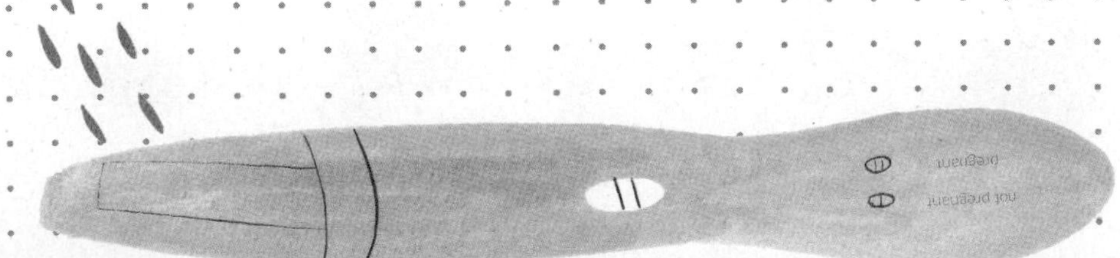
pregnant
not pregnant

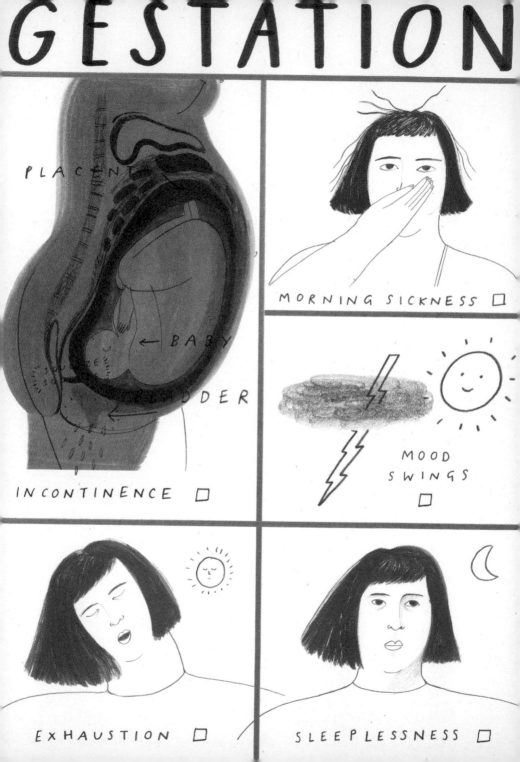

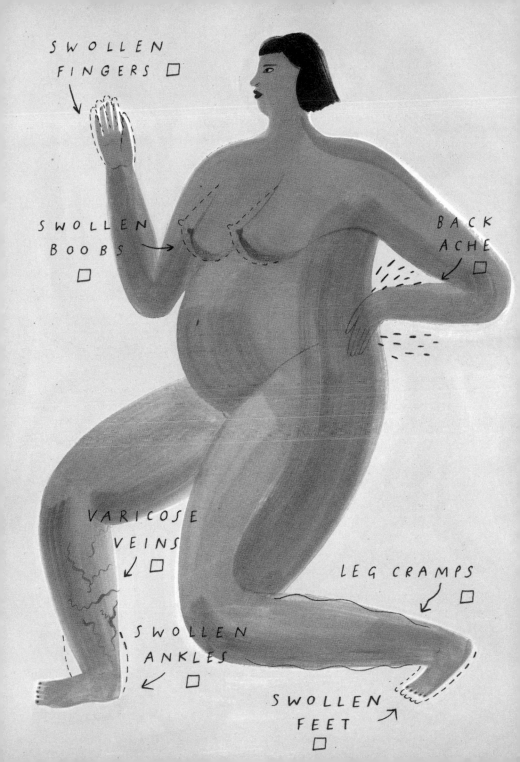

A NUTSHELL RETROSPECTIVE PREGNANCY DIARY

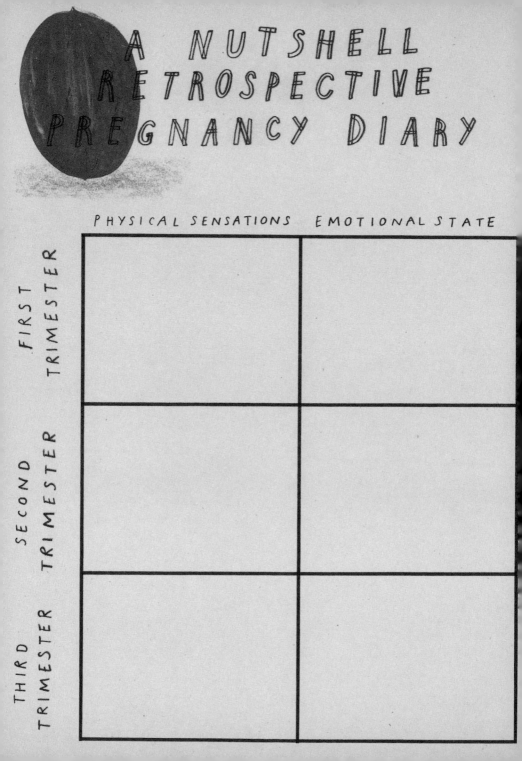

PHYSICAL SENSATIONS   EMOTIONAL STATE

FIRST TRIMESTER

SECOND TRIMESTER

THIRD TRIMESTER

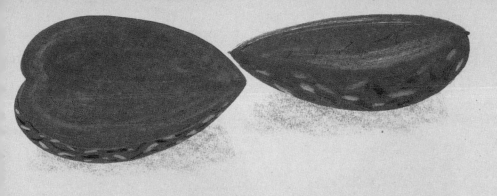

EXTERNAL EVENTS   ANYTHING ELSE?

VITAL STATISTICS

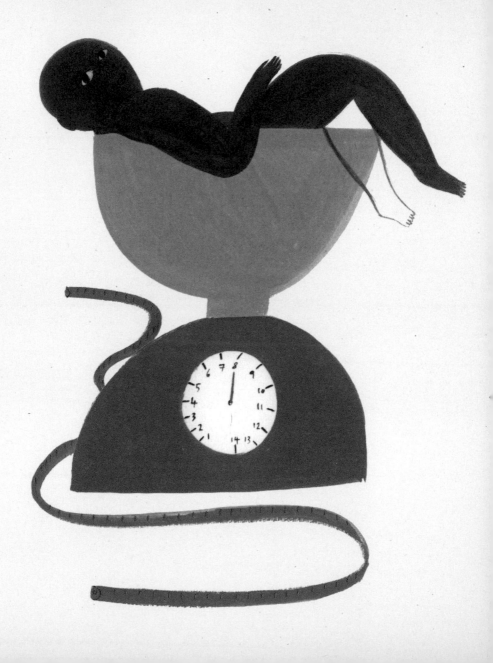

TIME of BIRTH
_____

DATE of BIRTH
_____

METHOD of DELIVERY
_____

WEIGHT_____

HEIGHT _____

GENDER _____

HAIR ?_____

The Birth

write the birth story of your baby in as much detail as you can

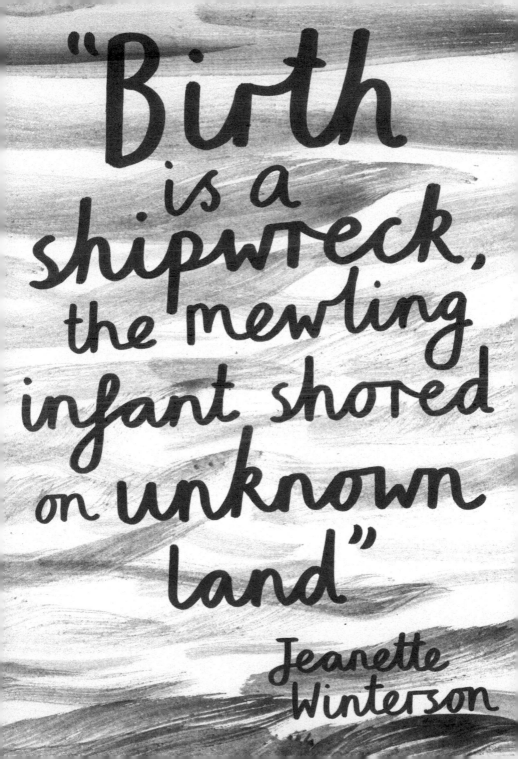

"Birth is a shipwreck, the mewling infant shored on unknown land"

Jeanette Winterson

Draw your little one awake

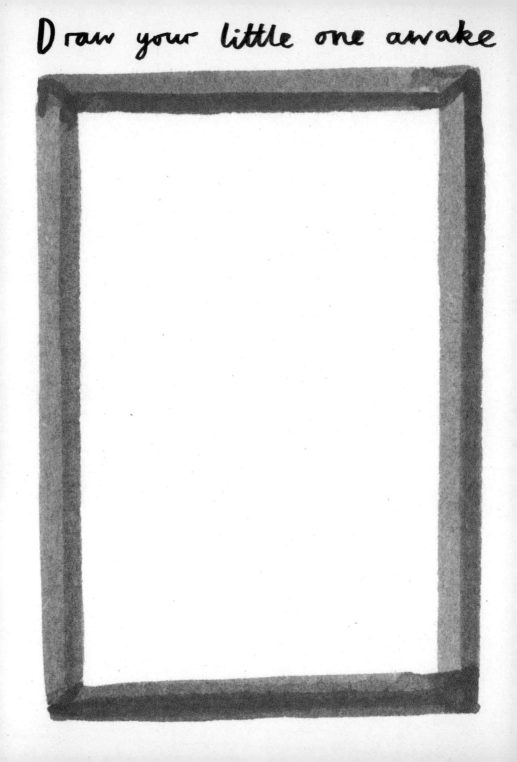

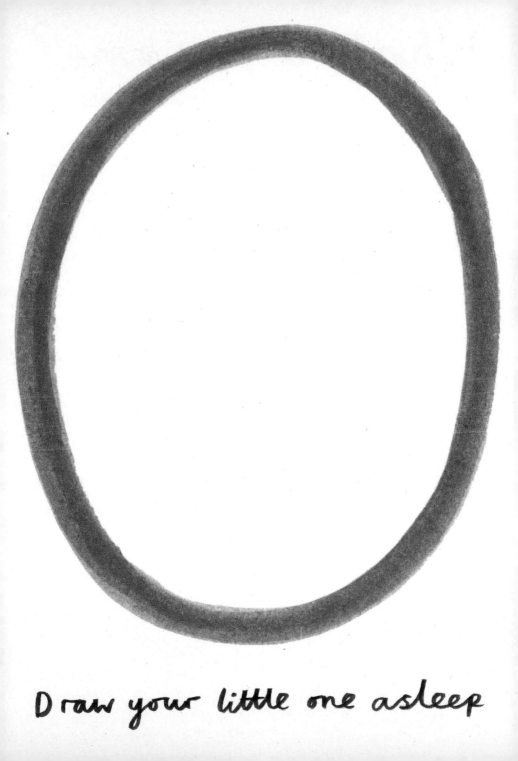

Draw your little one asleep

What's in a name?

How did you choose your baby's name?
Do you know the story behind your own name?

Any near misses?

Fill in the name tags with any names you nearly went for.

WISE N...
Dara, H...
Ethan,
Socrate...

Delia, Althea,
Heather, Iris,
June, Jupiter,
Laurel, Opal

TOP
1000
BABY
NAMES

MYSTICAL
NAMES

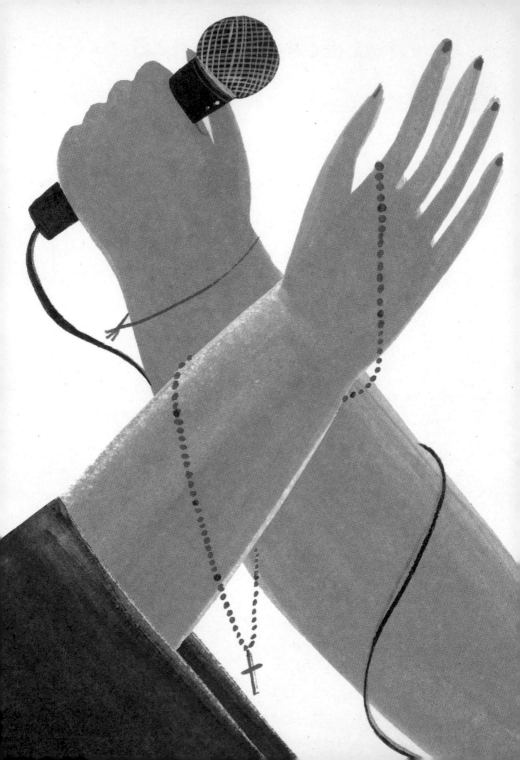

"I sometimes think I was born to live up to my name. How could I be anything else but what I am having been *named* **Madonna**? I would have either ended up as a nun or this"

Madonna

Early Days

What emotions did you experience in the first days of motherhood? What did you feel when you first saw your little one?

Don't hold back!

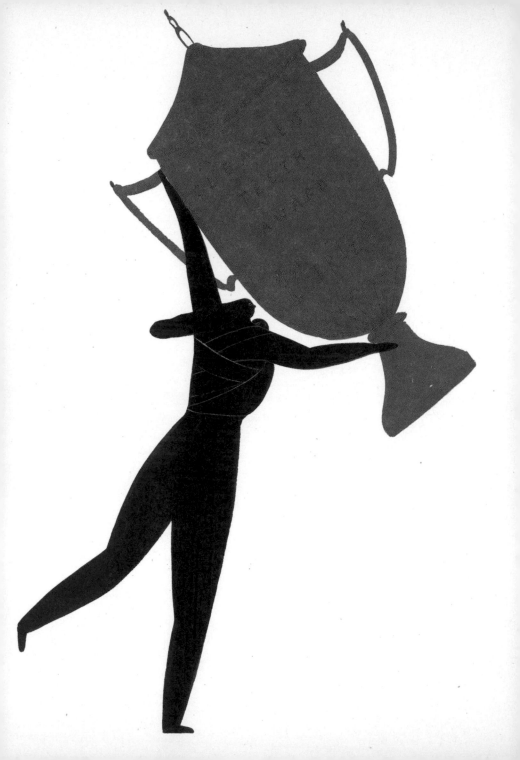

TODAY I MANAGED TO...

- ✓ GET OUT OF BED
- HAVE A SHOWER
- BE NICE TO MY PARTNER
- GO TO THE TOILET
- GET MYSELF DRESSED
- BRUSH MY TEETH
- MAKE MYSELF A SANDWICH
- NOT CRY
- TALK TO ANOTHER HUMAN BEING
- LEAVE THE HOUSE

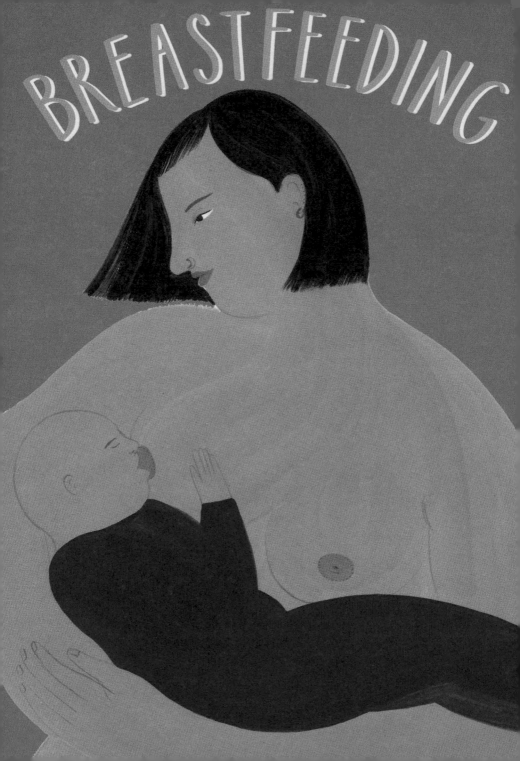

Write your experiences of breastfeeding or non-breastfeeding
What are your emotional and physical responses
to the expectations and realities of breastfeeding?

Sleeep

MONTHS

AVERAGE HOURS SLEPT	1	2	3	4	5
1					
2					
3					
4					
5					
6					
7					
8					

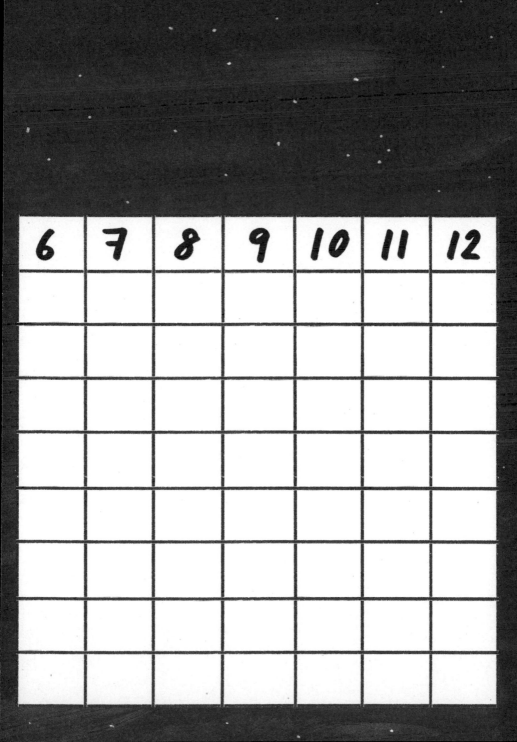

6	7	8	9	10	11	12

ADVICE

What was the best and worst advice you were given after the birth of your baby?

Describe your little one in the early days

What are
they like now?

Apples and trees

write a list of traits you see in your child.
What do you most relate to?

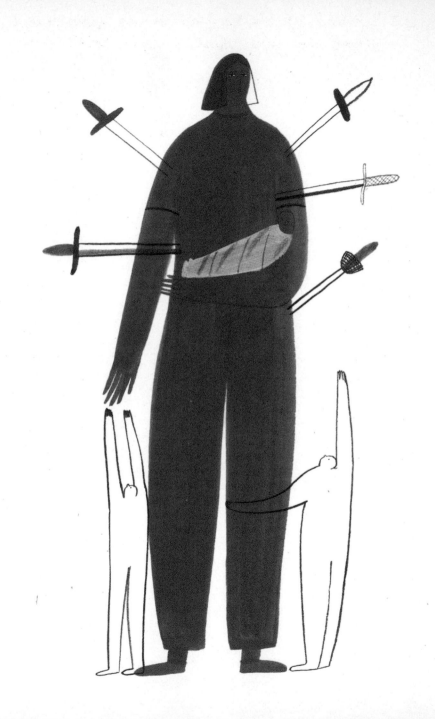

"what fabrications
they are, mothers.
Scarecrows, wax dolls
for us to stick our pins into,
crude diagrams.
we deny them an
existence of their own,
we make them up to
suit ourselves,
our own hungers,
our own wishes,
our own deficiencies"

Margaret Atwood
The Blind Assassin

my mother, myself

Write about your relationship with your mother.
Write about all the things you believe she did right and wrong.

Draw a picture of your mum

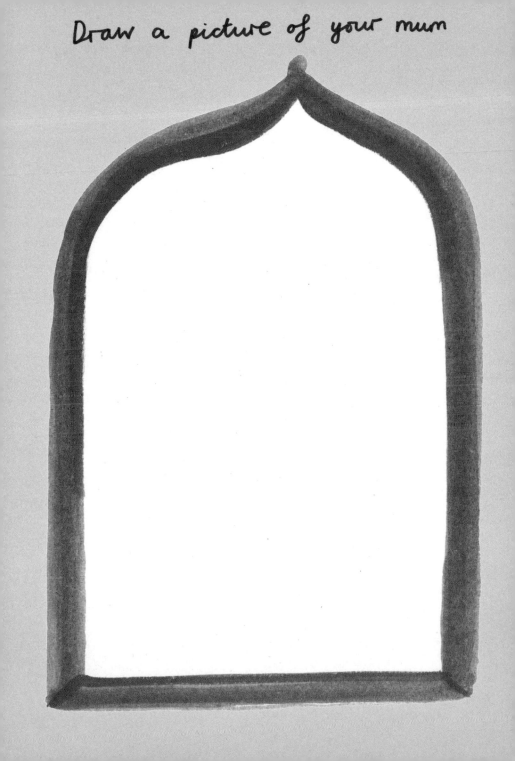

What kind of mother do you want to be?

What mistakes
do you want
to avoid?

What values do you want to pass on to your children?

PROMISES
TO MAKE FOR YOUR BABY

Which have you made? Which can you keep?
What is really important to you?

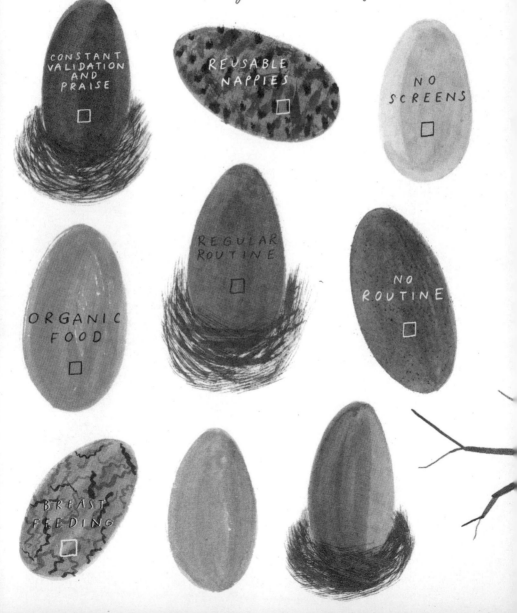

CONSTANT VALIDATION AND PRAISE ☐

REUSABLE NAPPIES ☐

NO SCREENS ☐

REGULAR ROUTINE ☐

ORGANIC FOOD ☐

NO ROUTINE ☐

BREAST FEEDING ☐

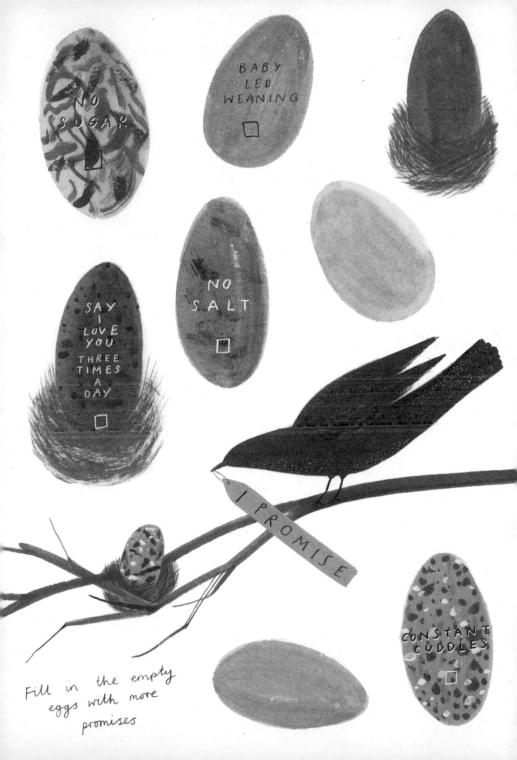

NO SUGAR

BABY LED WEANING

NO SALT

SAY I LOVE YOU THREE TIMES A DAY

I PROMISE

CONSTANT CUDDLES

Fill in the empty eggs with more promises

Write and draw all of your hopes and dreams for your little one.

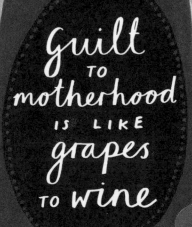

guilt TO motherhood IS LIKE grapes TO wine

Fay Weldon

What do you feel most anxious about?

What makes you feel like you're doing it all wrong?

Describe a
moment
in which you felt
you failed.

Try to describe it again through the eyes of a stranger

"The idea that you sacrifice everything for your children - it's a LOAD of RUBBISH... it's elevating the child at the expense of the MOTHER

It's like your Life is not valid except in fulfilling this child's needs.

What about all
your needs,
your desires,
your wants,
your problems?"

Marina Carr

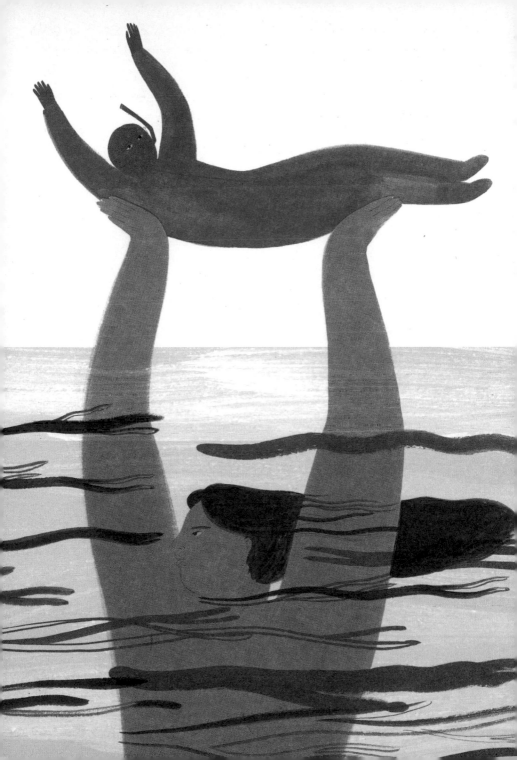

write your hopes and ambitions for yourself - the ones that
you have had to let go of and the ones you must always hold onto.

Lost dreams

Dreams that must never be lost

Write all your feelings about your partner.

what do you love, what drives you crazy?

united front

How similar / different are your parenting priorities from your partner's?

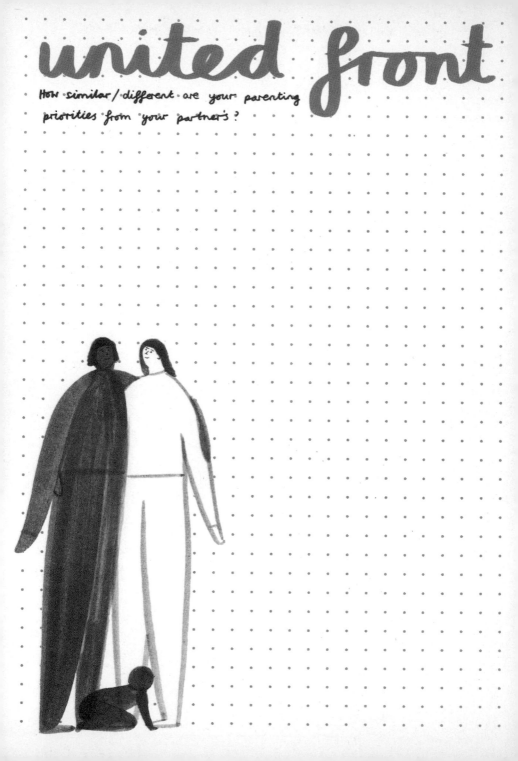

What kind of upbringing did he/she have?
How did it differ from yours? Where is your common ground?

WORK LIFE BALANCE

fill the scales with all the elements in both
life and work that you are
responsible for.

WORK

Draw them in proportion to the mental space they require.

LIFE

Which side is heavier?

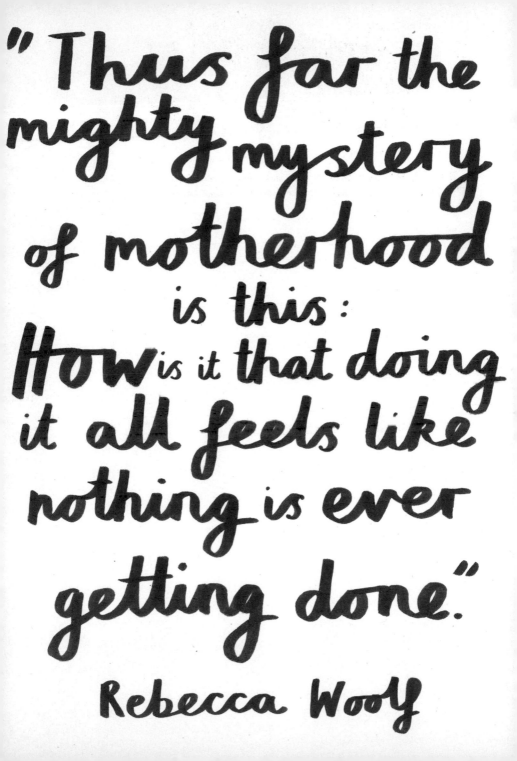

"Thus far the mighty mystery of motherhood is this: **How** is it that doing it all feels like nothing is ever getting done."

Rebecca Woolf

Domestic Drudgery

How are the domestic tasks shared between you and your partner? What are the daily chores that really drive you up the wall?

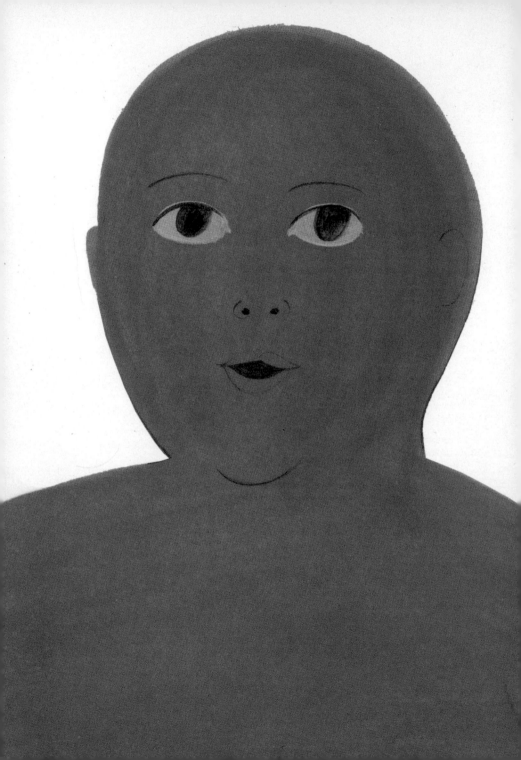

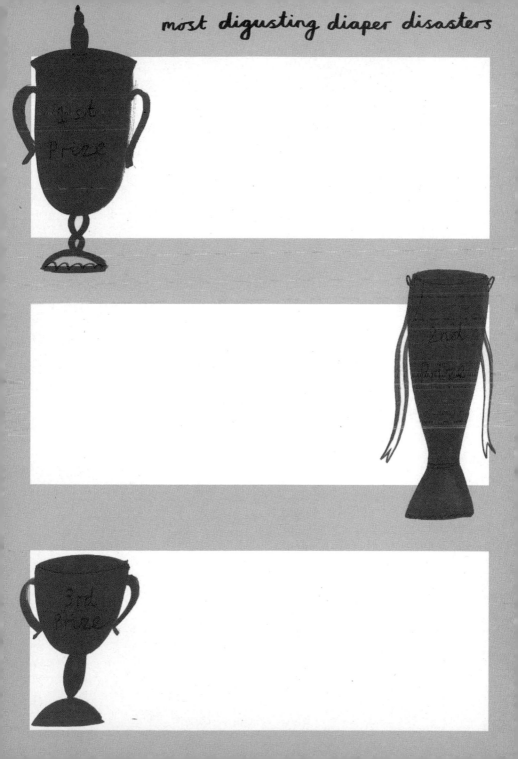

STITCHES
sketches
SCARS

write how you feel about your body post-pregnancy.

use this space to draw your body

SEX

Has childbirth changed the way feel you about sex?
Has your connection to your body or your desirability changed?

women vs women

We are often too hard on ourselves and therefore other women. Take a break from the inner diatribe and write about what other mums around you are doing RIGHT.

Describe some moments in which you felt admiration at the strength and resourcefulness of women around you.

Pick a stereotype

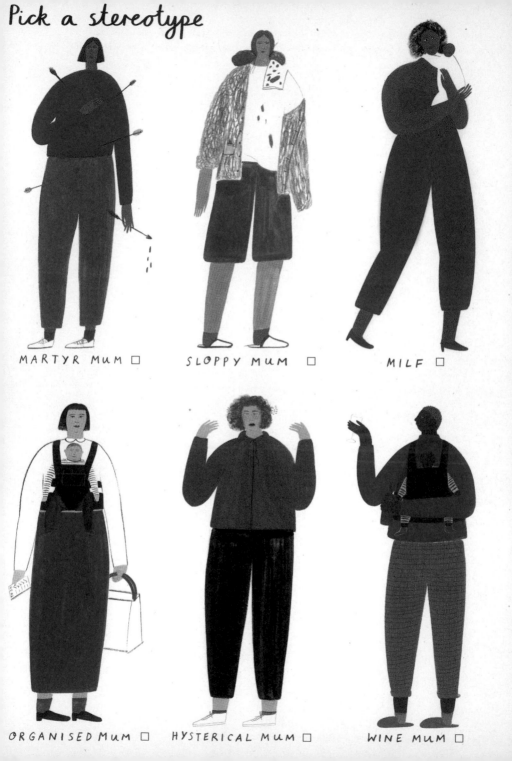

MARTYR MUM ☐

SLOPPY MUM ☐

MILF ☐

ORGANISED MUM ☐

HYSTERICAL MUM ☐

WINE MUM ☐

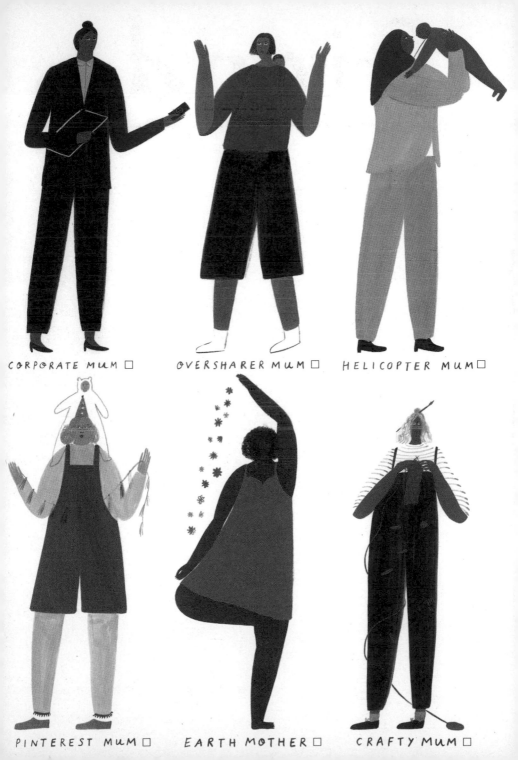

CORPORATE MUM ☐   OVERSHARER MUM ☐   HELICOPTER MUM ☐

PINTEREST MUM ☐   EARTH MOTHER ☐   CRAFTY MUM ☐

Friends

How did your friends respond when you became a mum?

Did you feel isolated
or supported ?

Did you make new friends?

STRESS!!!

when does it all feel too much?
what are your stress triggers?
what are your coping strategies?

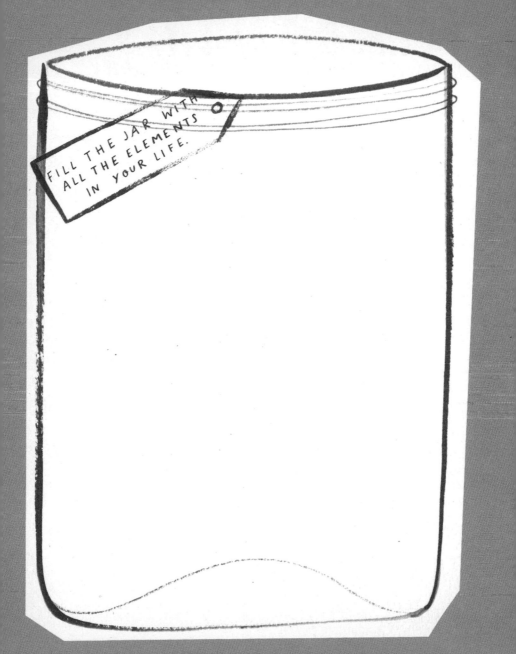

FILL THE JAR WITH ALL THE ELEMENTS IN YOUR LIFE.

What takes up a lot of headspace? What doesn't? What elements would you like to reduce? What elements would you like to create space for?

MINDFULNESS

BREAK YOUR FOCUS AWAY
FROM YOUR IMMEDIATE SITUATION
AND FOCUS ON YOUR SURROUNDINGS.
CAN YOU SPOT 5 ROUND OBJECTS?
CAN YOU HEAR 3 DIFFERENT NOISES?

TRY TO FEEL PRESENT IN THE MOMENT.

STOP WHAT YOU'RE DOING,
CLOSE YOUR EYES AND
FOCUS ON YOUR BREATH.
TAKE FIVE DEEP BREATHS.
IN AND OUT.

SIT OR LIE DOWN ON THE FLOOR.
CONNECT WITH YOUR BODY AND
FEEL THE WAY IT IS ROOTED TO THE FLOOR.

CLENCH EACH MUSCLE INDIVIDUALLY

AND THEN RELEASE.

TAKE A WALK.
EVEN IF YOU CAN BARELY
PUT ON YOUR SHOES, CHANGING YOUR
SURROUNDINGS AND CONNECTING WITH
NATURE ALWAYS GIVES YOU A BOOST

BE KIND TO YOURSELF!

THERE'S NO WAY TO GET IT RIGHT
SO DON'T BEAT YOURSELF UP FOR
GETTING IT WRONG SOMETIMES.

GRATITUDE

Take a moment to write a
list of all the things that
are good in your life.

"For every ailment under the sun,
There is a remedy, or there is none,
If there be one, try to find it,
If there be none, never mind it."
Mother Goose

"My children cause me the MOST exquisite suffering of which I have any experience. It is the suffering of ambivalence: the MURDEROUS alternation between BITTER resentment and RAW EDGED nerves and BLISSFUL gratification and tenderness"

Adrienne Rich

magical moment

low point

STRONG

write down a list of times in your life
in which you've had to find inner strength

A woman is like a teabag. You can't tell how strong she is until you put her in hot water "

Eleanor Roosevelt

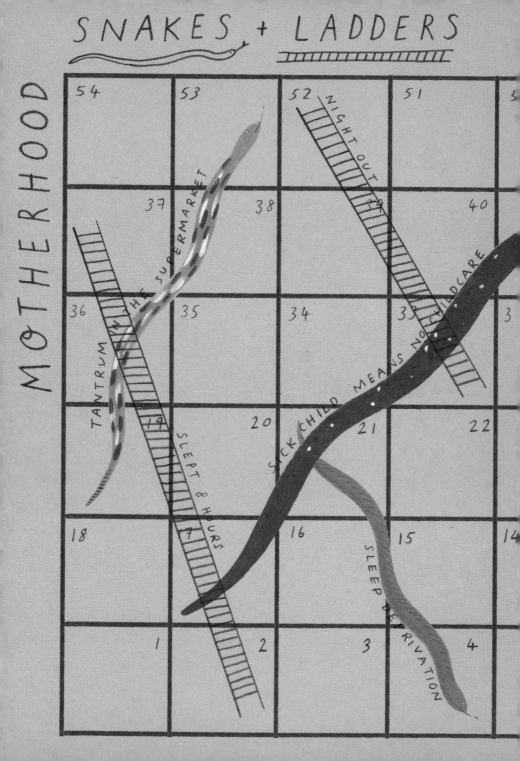

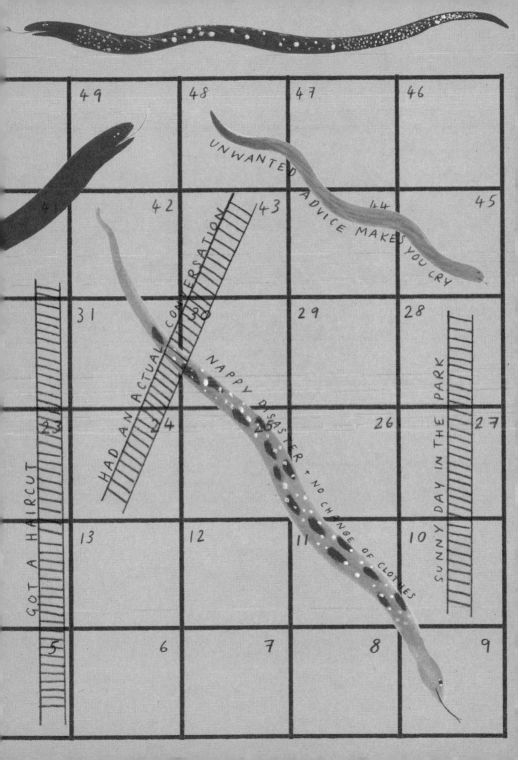

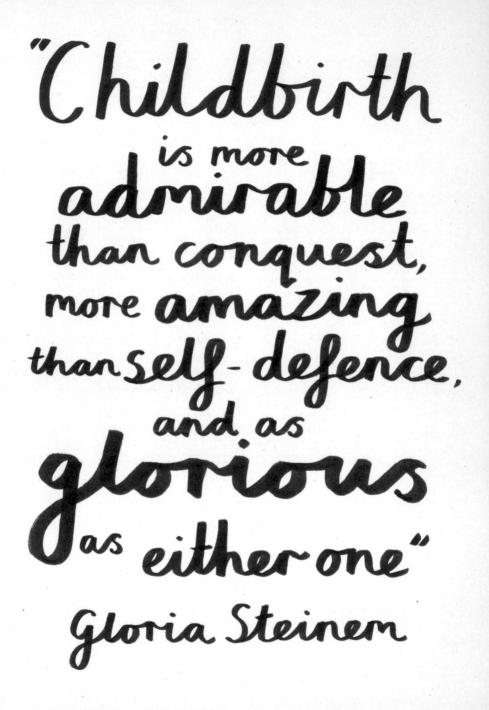

"Childbirth is more admirable than conquest, more amazing than self-defence, and as glorious as either one"

Gloria Steinem

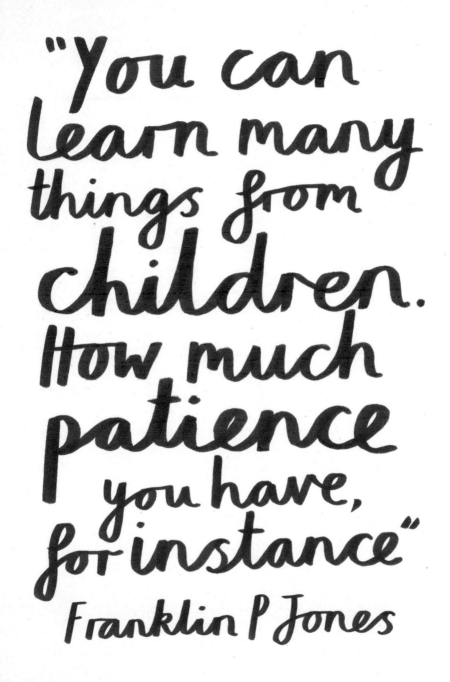

Motherlode

Published by Cicada Books Limited

Illustrated by Georgie McAusland
Text by Ziggy Hanaor

British Library Cataloguing-in-Publication Data.

A CIP record for this book is available from the British Library.
ISBN: 978-1-908714-58-9

Cicada Books Limited
48 Burghley Road
London
NW5 1UE
www.cicadabooks.co.uk

Printed in Poland